The Beauty of Witchcraft

medieval pharmacy and healing, Vol. II

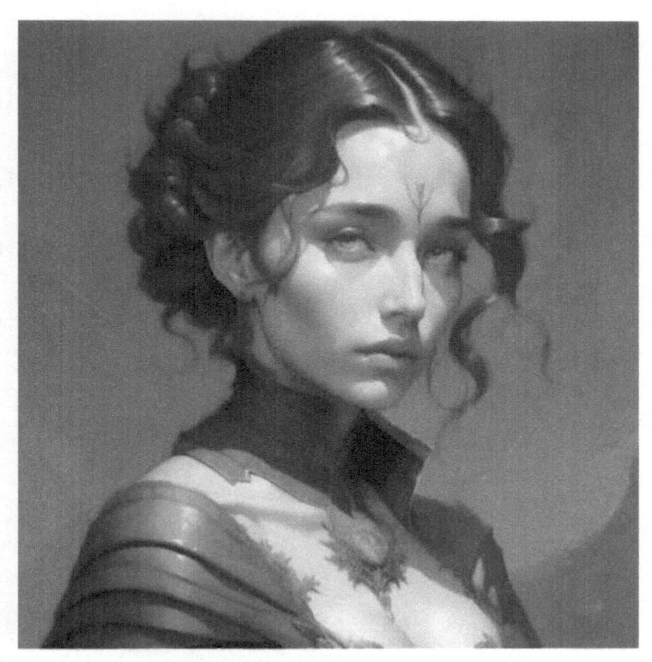

Table of Contents

Intro..6

400 Years of Persecution Mania............................8

   15th Century Persecution...........................10

   16th century persecution in Germany, Switzerland and France, and Scotland............13

   17th century persecution in Germany, Switzerland, France, and Scotland.................16

   18th century persecution in Germany, Switzerland, France, and Scotland.................19

   19th Century: Not even Apologies....................22

Art of Healing...24

   Witches' Art of Healing during the 15th Century....................................24

   15th Century Science?...............................27

   Witches' Art of Healing during the 16th Century....................................29

   16th Century Science?...............................32

   Witches' Art of Healing during the 17th Century....................................34

   17th Century Science?...............................37

   Witches' Art of Healing during the 18th Century....................................39

   18th Century Science?...............................42

Witchcraft Legacy..44

   Liquids...44

   Special Healing Brews...............................46

      German Specifics.................................49

      Swiss Specifics.................................51

French Specifics...53
Scottish Specifics..55
Cultural Differences between Witches in Germany, Switzerland, France and Scotland........................57
Witches Brews and Modern Day Medicine.........60
Witchcraft vs. today's Pharmaceutical Industry...62
Skin in the Game...64

Intro

The perception and treatment of witches varied throughout different regions and time periods, most of those accused and persecuted as witches were women, and their practices often revolved around folk medicine and healing.

During the Middle Ages, the belief in witchcraft was widespread across Europe. The Church played a significant role in shaping the perception of witches, viewing them as practitioners of magic who made pacts with the devil. This belief was reinforced by texts such as the Malleus Maleficarum (Hexenhammer), a notorious manual on witch-hunting published in the late 15th century.

Accusations of witchcraft were often driven by a combination of religious, social, and cultural factors. In times of crisis, such as outbreaks of disease, natural disasters, or crop failures, individuals were quick to look for scapegoats, and vulnerable women—often healers or wise women—were frequently targeted. Their knowledge of herbal remedies, midwifery, and folk practices was misunderstood and seen as evidence of dark supernatural powers.

It's important to note that the image of the witch as an evil, malevolent figure was largely a construct of the time. In reality, many of those accused were likely ordinary people practicing traditional forms of healing and folk magic. Their knowledge of herbs and remedies often made them respected figures within their communities. However, the widespread fear and suspicion surrounding witchcraft led to numerous trials, persecutions, and, tragically, executions.

Today, there is a growing recognition and reevaluation of the historical treatment of witches. Scholars and historians are working to dispel the misconceptions and myths surrounding witchcraft, highlighting the social and cultural dynamics at play during the medieval period.

400 Years of Persecution Mania

The persecution of individuals accused of witchcraft in Europe took place over a considerable span of time, but it primarily occurred between the early 15th and late 18th century A.D. This period is often referred to as the "Early Modern Witch Hunts" or the "European Witch Craze."

The exact starting point of the witch hunts is difficult to pinpoint precisely, as beliefs in witchcraft and sporadic persecutions existed prior to the 15th century. However, the intensity and scale of the witch hunts increased significantly from the late 15th century onward.

The height of the witch hunts is generally considered to be the 16th and 17th centuries. During this time, numerous witch trials were conducted throughout Europe, resulting in the execution of thousands of people, mostly women. The exact number of victims is uncertain, but estimates range from tens of thousands to hundreds of thousands.

It's worth noting that the intensity of the witch hunts varied across different regions. Certain areas, such as parts of Germany, Switzerland, France, and Scotland, experienced particularly widespread and brutal persecutions. Other regions, such as parts of Italy and Spain, saw relatively fewer witch trials.

By the 18th century, attitudes towards witchcraft began to shift. Skepticism grew, and legal reforms were implemented in some areas, leading to a decline in witch trials. The Enlightenment period played a significant role in challenging traditional beliefs in witchcraft and fostering a more rational and skeptical approach.

15th Century Persecution

The persecution of witches in Germany, Switzerland, France, and Scotland during the 15th century underwent significant developments and variations in each region.

While the witch hunts of the 16th and 17th centuries are generally considered the peak of persecution, there were notable developments during the 15th century that laid the groundwork for the later witch trials.

The Malleus Maleficarum: One of the most influential texts on witchcraft, the Malleus Maleficarum (Hexenhammer), was written by Heinrich Kramer and Jacob Sprenger and published in 1487. It served as a guidebook for identifying, prosecuting, and eradicating witchcraft. The Malleus Maleficarum presented a detailed account of witches, their alleged practices, and the methods to be used in their trials and interrogations. This text had a profound impact on shaping attitudes toward witchcraft and contributed to the increasing fear and paranoia surrounding witches.

Papal Bull Summis desiderantes affectibus: In 1484, Pope Innocent VIII issued the papal bull Summis desiderantes affectibus, which empowered inquisitors Heinrich Kramer and Jacob Sprenger to investigate and prosecute individuals accused of witchcraft in the German states. This papal endorsement lent authority to the witch trials and reinforced the belief in the existence of witches and their connection to demonic forces.

Increased Fear and Social Tensions: The 15th century witnessed various social, political, and religious upheavals, including the Protestant Reformation, the Hussite Wars, and the consolidation of centralized power. These disruptions, coupled with natural disasters and epidemics, created an atmosphere of fear and uncertainty. The belief in witches as malevolent agents who caused harm, illness, and misfortune gained traction as people sought explanations for the crises they faced.

Local Trials and Precedents: Prior to the 15th century, localized cases of witchcraft accusations and trials occurred sporadically across Europe. While not as widespread or systematic as in later periods, these local trials served as precursors and contributed to the evolving understanding and perception of witches and witchcraft.

It is important to note that while these developments in the 15th century laid the groundwork for the witch hunts that followed, they did not represent a full-scale witch craze. The intensity and scale of the witch trials increased significantly in the 16th and 17th centuries, with different regions experiencing different levels of persecution.

16th century persecution in Germany, Switzerland and France, and Scotland

Germany

During the 16th century, the witch trials in Germany reached a peak of intensity. Witchcraft was seen as a significant threat, both religiously and socially. The printing and widespread circulation of the Malleus Maleficarum (1487) by Heinrich Kramer and Jacob Sprenger contributed to the growing fear of witchcraft. Accusations and trials became more common, especially in regions like the Rhineland, Swabia, and Franconia. Women were the primary targets, accused of engaging in malevolent magic, causing harm, and forming pacts with the devil. The use of torture to extract confessions was prevalent, and the accused were often executed by burning at the stake.

Switzerland

In Switzerland, the witch hunts also gained momentum during the 16th century. The intensity of persecution varied across different cantons. Regions like Basel and Zurich witnessed more active witch trials. The accused were primarily women, though men were not exempt from accusations. Charges included causing illness, misfortune, or engaging in diabolical practices.

Torture was frequently employed to extract confessions. The preferred method of execution was burning at the stake.

France

In France, the 16th century saw fluctuations in the intensity of witchcraft persecution. During the late 16th century, under the reign of King Henry IV and his regents, witch trials were relatively infrequent. However, during the reign of Louis XIII, the witch hunts intensified, particularly in regions such as Lorraine, Alsace, and Burgundy. Accusations against witches were driven by religious and social tensions. Both women and men from various social backgrounds were targeted. Charges included causing harm, making pacts with the devil, and practicing malevolent magic. Burning at the stake was the most common form of execution.

Scotland

Scotland experienced a notable period of witchcraft persecution during the late 16th and early 17th centuries. The Scottish witch trials were characterized by a distinct legal framework known as the "witchcraft acts." The Witchcraft Act of 1563 and subsequent revisions provided a legal basis for prosecuting witches. Women were the primary victims of accusations, though men were also targeted. Charges ranged from causing harm and making pacts with the devil to practicing malevolent magic. Notable cases, such as the North Berwick witch trials of the 1590s, involved accusations of witchcraft against individuals associated with King James VI. Burning at the stake was the primary method of execution, although other forms of punishment were also used.

17th century persecution in Germany, Switzerland, France, and Scotland

Germany

In Germany, the witch hunts continued to be widespread and intense during the 17th century. The persecution was fueled by religious and social tensions, as well as the prevailing belief in the existence of witches. Witch trials were particularly prevalent in regions like Bavaria, where the Witch Hunts of Bamberg (1626-1631) and the Witch Hunts of Würzburg (1626-1631) resulted in thousands of executions. Women remained the primary targets, accused of practicing malevolent magic, causing harm, and consorting with the devil. Torture was often employed to extract confessions, and the accused were commonly executed by burning at the stake.

Switzerland

In Switzerland, the 17th century witnessed a continuation of the witch hunts, although with varying intensity across different cantons. Witch trials were more frequent in regions like Zurich, Lucerne, and Bern. The accused, mostly women, were charged with engaging in witchcraft, causing harm, and making pacts with the devil. Torture was employed to elicit confessions, and the preferred method of execution remained burning at the stake.

France
The persecution of witches in France during the 17th century saw a gradual decline compared to the previous century. While sporadic cases of witchcraft accusations and trials still occurred, the intensity decreased, and the overall fervor diminished. This shift was partly influenced by a growing skepticism towards witchcraft and an increasing influence of Enlightenment ideas. However, certain regions, such as Lorraine and Alsace, still experienced notable witch trials during this period, with women primarily being accused. Burning at the stake remained the primary method of execution.

Scotland
In Scotland, the 17th century marked a continuation of witchcraft persecution, particularly during the reign of King James VI (later James I of England). The North Berwick witch trials in the late 16th century, which implicated individuals close to the king, further fueled the witch hunts. The Witchcraft Act of 1563 continued to provide the legal framework for prosecutions. Accusations and trials increased, and women were the main targets. Charges included causing harm, practicing malevolent magic, and making pacts with the devil. Although burning at the stake remained a

common method of execution, other forms of punishment, such as hanging, were also employed.

It's important to note that the intensity and frequency of witch trials varied within these regions, and local circumstances, beliefs, and legal systems played significant roles in shaping the dynamics of persecution.

18th century persecution in Germany, Switzerland, France, and Scotland

During the 18th century, the persecution of witches in Germany, Switzerland, France, and Scotland began to decline significantly. Enlightenment ideas, growing skepticism, and changes in legal and social attitudes contributed to the diminishing intensity of witch trials.

Germany
By the 18th century, the witch hunts in Germany had largely subsided. The influence of Enlightenment thinkers and legal reforms played a crucial role in changing attitudes towards witchcraft. Authorities became more skeptical of supernatural explanations, and fewer witch trials took place. The use of torture to extract confessions was curtailed, and there was a shift towards more rational and evidence-based approaches in legal proceedings.

Switzerland
In Switzerland, the 18th century saw a significant decline in witch trials. The influence of the Enlightenment and legal reforms contributed to a more rational and skeptical approach. The belief in witchcraft gradually waned, and authorities

became less inclined to pursue accusations of witchcraft. The focus shifted away from supernatural explanations, and the persecution of witches became less common.

France
France experienced a notable decline in witchcraft persecution during the 18th century. The Enlightenment ideas, which emphasized reason and skepticism, had a profound impact on changing attitudes towards witchcraft. The belief in witchcraft diminished, and the legal framework for witch trials was gradually dismantled. Public sentiment turned against witch hunts, and fewer cases were pursued. The last recorded execution for witchcraft in France took place in 1745.

Scotland
In Scotland, the 18th century witnessed a significant decline in witch trials and persecutions. The Enlightenment era brought about a shift in intellectual and cultural attitudes, which led to increased skepticism regarding the existence of witches and witchcraft. The Witchcraft Act of 1735, which repealed the earlier witchcraft acts, signaled a change in legal perspectives. This act made it more challenging to prosecute individuals for witchcraft, resulting in a decline in witch trials.

Overall, the 18th century marked a turning point in the persecution of witches in these regions. The influence of the Enlightenment, changing social attitudes, and legal reforms contributed to a decline in witch trials and a more rational and skeptical approach to the subject.

19th Century: Not even Apologies

The 19th century did not see formal apologies for the persecution of individuals accused of witchcraft during the earlier centuries.

During the 19th century, societies were going through significant changes due to industrialization, urbanization, and political transformations. The focus of public attention shifted away from the witch trials of previous centuries, and there were other pressing issues to contend with. The Enlightenment ideas of reason, skepticism, and individual rights that had contributed to the decline of witch trials also brought about changes in societal perspectives.

However, it is worth noting that in the modern era, there have been efforts to reevaluate and acknowledge the historical injustice and suffering experienced by those accused and persecuted as witches. Scholars, historians, and organizations have worked to raise awareness about the persecution, challenge stereotypes, and foster a better understanding of the social, cultural, and gender dynamics that played a role in the witch hunts.

While formal apologies may not have been issued specifically for the witch trials of the past, there have been broader movements toward reconciliation and recognizing historical injustices in various contexts. These efforts aim to promote understanding, healing, and the prevention of similar injustices in the future.

Art of Healing

Witches' Art of Healing during the 15th Century

During the 15th century, witches' healing abilities were perceived in different ways, depending on the region and cultural context.

Germany
In Germany, witches' healing abilities were often viewed with suspicion and fear. While some accused witches were believed to possess healing powers, these abilities were often overshadowed by the prevailing perception of witches as practitioners of harmful magic. The healing powers attributed to witches were sometimes seen as evidence of their involvement in malevolent practices rather than genuine acts of healing.

Switzerland
In Switzerland, the perception of witches' healing abilities was mixed. Accused witches were believed to possess both harmful and healing magic. While some witches were feared for their ability to cause harm, others were recognized for their knowledge of herbal remedies and practical healing techniques. These healers, often referred to

as wise women, were sought after by their communities for their healing services.

France
In France, witches' healing abilities were often met with suspicion and skepticism. Accused witches were believed to possess supernatural powers associated with both harmful and healing magic. While some witches were reputed to have healing skills, their practices were often viewed as supernatural and potentially dangerous. The line between healing and harmful magic was blurred, and witches were sometimes accused of using their powers for malevolent purposes.

Scotland
In Scotland, witches' healing abilities were recognized and sought after by the community. Cunning folk or wise women accused of witchcraft were respected for their knowledge of herbal remedies, midwifery, and practical healing techniques. These healers played an important role in their communities, offering assistance in childbirth, remedies for ailments, and other healing services. However, during the witch trials, their healing abilities were sometimes distorted and used as evidence against them.

It's important to note that the perception of witches' healing abilities during the 15th century was often influenced by social and cultural beliefs, as well as prevailing attitudes towards witchcraft. While some individuals accused of witchcraft may have genuinely practiced healing arts, their abilities were often conflated with superstitions, fears, and misconceptions surrounding witchcraft.

15th Century Science?

During the 15th century, the activities and practices associated with witches would not be considered scientific in the modern sense, as the understanding and methods of science were quite different at that time.

The 15th century marked the transition from the Middle Ages to the Renaissance, and scientific inquiry was influenced by medieval scholasticism and the prevailing Aristotelian worldview. Science during this period relied heavily on deductive reasoning, authoritative texts, and established beliefs rather than empirical observation and experimentation.

Witchcraft, as understood in the 15th century, was often associated with occult practices, supernatural beliefs, and magic. The activities attributed to witches, such as spells, divination, or the use of potions, were considered outside the realm of scientific inquiry. They were often associated with superstition and viewed as conflicting with the dominant religious and intellectual frameworks of the time.

It's important to consider that the concept of scientific research as we understand it today, with its emphasis on systematic observation, experimentation, and the accumulation of empirical evidence, was not prevalent during the 15th century.

Witches' Art of Healing during the 16th Century

During the 16th century, witches' healing abilities were perceived and interpreted differently across different regions and cultural contexts.

Germany
In Germany, the perception of witches' healing abilities was generally negative. Witches were often associated with harmful magic and seen as causing illness or misfortune. While some accused witches were believed to possess healing powers, these abilities were often overshadowed by the prevailing fear and suspicion surrounding witches. The healing practices attributed to witches were often considered as evidence of their involvement in malevolent activities rather than genuine acts of healing.

Switzerland
In Switzerland, the perception of witches' healing abilities during the 16th century was mixed. Accused witches were believed to possess both harmful and healing powers. Some witches were feared for their ability to cause harm, while others were sought after for their knowledge of herbal remedies and practical healing techniques. Wise women or folk healers, accused of witchcraft, were

respected for their healing skills but were often persecuted due to the association of their practices with malevolent magic.

France
In France, witches' healing abilities were often met with skepticism and suspicion. While some witches were believed to have healing powers, their practices were often seen as supernatural and potentially dangerous. The line between healing and harmful magic was blurred, and witches were sometimes accused of using their abilities for malevolent purposes. The prevailing perception of witches during this period was that they possessed supernatural powers associated with both healing and harmful magic.

Scotland
In Scotland, witches' healing abilities were recognized and sought after by the community. Cunning folk or wise women accused of witchcraft were respected for their knowledge of herbal remedies, midwifery, and practical healing techniques. They played a vital role in their communities, offering assistance in childbirth, remedies for ailments, and other healing services. However, during the witch trials, their healing abilities were often distorted and used as evidence against them.

It's important to note that the perception of witches' healing abilities during the 16th century was influenced by cultural beliefs, religious doctrines, and the prevailing fears surrounding witchcraft. The understanding of healing powers attributed to witches varied, and the same practices and abilities could be interpreted positively or negatively depending on the context.

16th Century Science?

During the 16th century, the understanding and practice of science were significantly different from what we consider scientific today. The prevailing worldview was still heavily influenced by religious and philosophical beliefs, and the scientific methods we rely on, such as systematic observation, experimentation, and hypothesis testing, were not yet fully established.

Witches, as they were understood during that period, were often associated with supernatural and occult practices. Their activities were considered outside the realm of scientific inquiry, as they involved elements of magic, divination, and beliefs in the supernatural. The practices attributed to witches, such as casting spells, using charms, or performing rituals, were based on traditional knowledge, folk beliefs, and superstitions rather than empirical evidence or rigorous scientific investigation.

The development of modern scientific methods and the establishment of a more systematic approach to knowledge emerged during the Scientific Revolution in the 16th and 17th centuries. This period marked a significant shift in scientific inquiry, embracing empirical observation, experimentation, and the development of theories based on evidence.

Therefore, while the activities and practices associated with witches during the 16th century may have involved various forms of knowledge and experimentation, they would not align with the scientific research as understood today.

Witches' Art of Healing during the 17th Century

During the 17th century, the perception and understanding of witches' healing abilities continued to evolve, influenced by the prevailing religious, social, and cultural beliefs of the time.

Germany

In Germany, the perception of witches' healing abilities during the 17th century varied. While some accused witches were believed to possess healing powers, these abilities were often overshadowed by the prevailing fear and suspicion surrounding witchcraft. Accused witches were generally associated with harmful magic and seen as causing illness or misfortune. The notion of witches as healers was sometimes regarded with skepticism, as their practices were often intertwined with accusations of malevolent activities.

Switzerland

In Switzerland, the perception of witches' healing abilities during the 17th century remained mixed. Accused witches were believed to possess both harmful and healing powers. Some witches were feared for their potential to inflict harm, while others were sought after for their knowledge of herbal remedies and practical healing techniques. However, the association of witches with malevolent magic often overshadowed their healing abilities, leading to the persecution of those accused of witchcraft.

France

In France, the perception of witches' healing abilities during the 17th century shifted towards a more negative view. Witches were increasingly associated with harmful practices, and their alleged healing powers were often disregarded or interpreted as part of their malevolent activities. Accused witches were believed to engage in harmful magic, causing illness, and making pacts with supernatural entities. The prevailing belief was that witches used their powers for nefarious purposes rather than genuine healing.

Scotland

In Scotland, the perception of witches' healing abilities during the 17th century remained relatively consistent with previous centuries. Cunning folk or wise women accused of witchcraft were recognized and sought after for their healing skills. They played a crucial role in providing remedies, midwifery services, and practical healing techniques to their communities. Despite the overall negative view of witchcraft, accused witches with healing abilities were often seen as valuable members of society.

It's important to note that the perception of witches' healing abilities during the 17th century was influenced by cultural beliefs, religious doctrines, and the prevailing fears surrounding witchcraft. While some accused witches may have genuinely practiced healing arts, their abilities were often conflated with superstitions, fears, and miscon-ceptions surrounding witchcraft.

17th Century Science?

The scientific methods and approaches that we recognize today were not yet fully developed or widely practiced during the 17th century.

In the 17th century, scientific inquiry was influenced by various factors, including religious beliefs, philosophical traditions, and limited access to knowledge and resources. The prevailing scientific worldview was still rooted in a mixture of ancient and medieval ideas, such as Aristotelianism and scholasticism.

Witches, as they were understood during that period, were often associated with supernatural and occult practices. The activities attributed to witches, such as spellcasting, divination, or the use of potions, were considered outside the realm of scientific inquiry. They were often associated with folk beliefs, superstitions, and occult knowledge that were separate from the emerging scientific discourse.

The scientific revolution, which brought about a significant shift in scientific methodology and understanding, occurred in the 16th and 17th centuries but primarily after this period. During that time, new scientific approaches, such as empirical observation, experimentation, and the development of scientific theories, emerged.

Witches' Art of Healing during the 18th Century

During the 18th century, the perception of witches' healing abilities continued to change, influenced by shifting cultural, social, and intellectual contexts.

Germany

In Germany, the 18th century witnessed a decline in the belief in witches' healing abilities. The influence of the Enlightenment and rational thinking led to a more skeptical approach to witchcraft and supernatural phenomena. The perception of witches shifted from practitioners of healing to individuals associated with superstition and irrationality. The prevailing attitude was increasingly skeptical of magical or supernatural healing powers, and folk healers or wise women were viewed with less reverence than in previous centuries.

Switzerland

In Switzerland, the 18th century saw a similar decline in the belief in witches' healing abilities. The influence of the Enlightenment, coupled with legal reforms and the spread of scientific knowledge, contributed to a more rational and skeptical outlook. The perception of witches as healers gave way to a diminishing belief in supernatural powers, and the emphasis shifted towards evidence-based medicine and scientific understanding. The role of folk healers diminished, and their practices were increasingly viewed as outdated or superstitious.

France
In France, the 18th century marked a significant decline in witchcraft persecution and the belief in witches' healing abilities. The Enlightenment ideals of reason, skepticism, and scientific progress played a crucial role in challenging superstitions and traditional beliefs. The influence of Enlightenment thinkers and the spread of scientific knowledge led to a more rational and scientific approach to healing. Traditional folk healers were marginalized as scientific medicine gained prominence.

Scotland
In Scotland, the 18th century witnessed a decline in witchcraft persecution and the belief in witches' healing abilities. The influence of the Enlightenment and the spread of scientific ideas led to a more rational and skeptical outlook. Folk healers, known as "cunning folk," gradually lost their authority as scientific medicine gained prominence. The focus shifted from traditional healing practices to evidence-based medicine and scientific understanding.

Overall, the 18th century marked a significant shift in the perception of witches' healing abilities. The influence of the Enlightenment, scientific progress, and rational thinking led to a decline in the belief in supernatural powers and a more skeptical approach to witchcraft and magical healing. Traditional folk healers were increasingly marginalized as scientific medicine gained prominence.

18th Century Science?

The research conducted by witches during the 18th century would not be considered scientific by the standards of that time or by today's scientific understanding. The scientific methods and approaches we recognize today were still in the process of development and had not fully matured during the 18th century.

During the 18th century, the Enlightenment brought about a significant shift in scientific thinking, emphasizing reason, evidence-based inquiry, and a more systematic approach to knowledge. Science during this period was increasingly influenced by empirical observation, experimentation, and the application of rational principles.

Witches, as understood during that period, were often associated with supernatural and occult practices. The activities attributed to witches, such as spellcasting, divination, or the use of potions, were considered outside the realm of scientific inquiry. They were associated with folk beliefs, superstitions, and practices that were separate from the emerging scientific discourse.

Scientific research in the 18th century was primarily carried out by natural philosophers and early scientists who adhered to the principles of empiricism and rationalism. They focused on systematic observation, experimentation, and the development of theories based on evidence. While the scientific landscape of the 18th century was in transition, it still followed a distinct methodological approach that distinguished it from the practices and beliefs associated with witchcraft.

Witchcraft Legacy

Liquids

There is no comprehensive list of liquids specifically attributed to witches, as the practices and beliefs associated with witchcraft varied across different cultures, regions, and historical periods. However, there were certain substances and concoctions that were commonly associated with witchcraft or used in magical rituals and remedies.

Flying Ointments: Flying ointments were believed to be used by witches to aid in their supposed ability to fly or have out-of-body experiences. These ointments often contained a mixture of herbs such as belladonna, mandrake, henbane, and other psychoactive plants, which were believed to induce hallucinations and altered states of consciousness.

Love Potions: Love potions were often associated with witches and magical practitioners. These potions were believed to have the power to influence the emotions or desires of individuals. They could be made using a variety of ingredients, including herbs, flowers, and sometimes exotic or rare substances.

Healing Brews: Witches, particularly those considered wise women or folk healers, were believed to possess knowledge of herbal remedies and medicinal potions. They would create various herbal brews and infusions using plants known for their healing properties. These brews were used to treat ailments and promote health.

Divination Elixirs: Witches and fortune-tellers were often associated with the practice of divination. They would use different liquids, such as water, oil, or ink, for scrying or other forms of divination. These substances were believed to have the ability to reveal hidden knowledge or insights into the future.

It's important to note that the historical understanding of witchcraft and the substances associated with it often involved a mix of folklore, superstition, and cultural beliefs. Many of these substances were considered part of magical or occult practices rather than scientifically proven remedies or potions.

Special Healing Brews

Details about the specific healing brews used by witches can vary depending on cultural beliefs, regional traditions, and historical periods. However, there were common ingredients and practices associated with herbal healing brews used by witches and folk healers.

Herbal Infusions: Witches and folk healers often relied on herbal infusions or teas made from various medicinal plants. Different plants were chosen based on their healing properties and intended effects. Commonly used herbs included chamomile, lavender, mint, rosemary, nettle, yarrow, and many others. These herbs were steeped in hot water to extract their medicinal properties and consumed as a tea or tonic.

Poultices and Compresses: Witches and folk healers would also create poultices or compresses using herbs and other ingredients. These poultices were typically made by grinding or mashing fresh or dried herbs and mixing them with water or other liquids to create a paste. The paste was then applied directly to the affected area of the body to alleviate pain, reduce inflammation, or promote healing.

Herbal Baths: Witches and folk healers often prescribed herbal baths for various purposes, such as relaxation, cleansing, and healing. A variety of herbs, flowers, or aromatic plants would be infused in hot water, and the person seeking healing would soak in the herbal bath. This was believed to promote relaxation, relieve muscle tension, and provide therapeutic benefits.

Herbal Tinctures and Extracts: Witches and folk healers also created concentrated herbal extracts and tinctures. These were made by soaking herbs in alcohol or vinegar over a period of time to extract their medicinal properties. The resulting liquid was then used in small doses as a remedy for specific ailments or as a general tonic for overall health.

Specific recipes and practices for creating healing brews varied among different cultures and individual healers. The selection of herbs, their proportions, and the specific methods of preparation often relied on traditional knowledge passed down through generations or personal experience of the healer.

Some remedies and ingredients used by witches and folk healers may not align with modern medical understanding or may have had limited efficacy. Historical healing practices were influenced by cultural beliefs, folklore, and traditional knowledge, and their effectiveness can vary greatly.

German Specifics

Herbal Knowledge: Witches and folk healers in Germany were known for their extensive knowledge of local plants and their healing properties. They would gather various herbs and flowers, both wild and cultivated, and incorporate them into their healing brews. Common medicinal plants used in German folk medicine included chamomile, yarrow, stinging nettle, calendula, valerian, and many others.

Traditional Recipes: German folk healing often relied on traditional recipes and formulations passed down through generations. These recipes involved specific combinations of herbs, roots, and other ingredients. Each remedy was believed to address specific ailments or promote general well-being. The precise recipes varied depending on the region and the preferences of individual healers.

Brewing Methods: Healing brews in Germany were often made as herbal infusions or decoctions. Herbal infusions involved pouring hot water over a mixture of herbs and allowing them to steep for a period of time. Decoctions, on the other hand, involved boiling the herbs in water to extract their medicinal properties. Both methods were used to create potent liquids that could be consumed as teas or tonics.

Local and Seasonal Ingredients: Witches and folk healers in Germany often utilized ingredients readily available in their local surroundings. They would gather herbs and plants growing in the region, taking advantage of their medicinal properties. Furthermore, seasonal availability played a role, as certain plants and flowers were collected and used at specific times of the year when they were believed to be most potent.

Ritual and Intention: The preparation of healing brews by witches often involved ritualistic practices and a focus on intention. It was believed that the healer's intentions and energy infused into the brew could enhance its healing properties. Rituals could involve chants, prayers, or other forms of invocation to empower the healing brews with their intended effects.

Swiss Specifics

Herbal Knowledge: Witches and folk healers in Switzerland were known for their understanding of local plants and their medicinal properties. They would gather a variety of herbs and plants, often found in the Swiss Alps and surrounding regions, for use in their healing brews. Common medicinal plants used in Swiss folk medicine included chamomile, sage, thyme, St. John's wort, yarrow, and others.

Traditional Formulations: Swiss folk healing relied on traditional formulations and recipes passed down through generations. These formulations involved specific combinations of herbs, roots, and other ingredients, with each remedy believed to address specific ailments or promote general well-being. The exact recipes varied depending on the region and the knowledge of individual healers.

Infusions and Decoctions: Witches and folk healers in Switzerland often prepared healing brews as infusions or decoctions. Infusions involved steeping herbs in hot water for a period of time, while decoctions involved boiling the herbs in water to extract their medicinal properties. Both methods were used to create potent liquids that could be consumed as teas or tonics.

Local and Alpine Ingredients: Witches and folk healers in Switzerland made use of ingredients available in their local environment, including those found in the Alpine regions. They gathered herbs and plants from the surrounding areas, taking advantage of their specific healing properties. This often included plants adapted to the Alpine climate, such as edelweiss, arnica, and gentian.

Ritual and Folklore: The preparation of healing brews in Switzerland often involved rituals and was imbued with folklore and traditional practices. The use of chants, prayers, or other ritualistic elements was believed to enhance the healing properties of the brews. Folklore and cultural beliefs surrounding the power of certain plants and rituals played a role in shaping the understanding of witches' healing abilities.

French Specifics

Herbal Knowledge: Witches and folk healers in France were known for their understanding of local plants and their medicinal properties. They would gather various herbs, flowers, and other botanical ingredients for use in their healing brews. Common medicinal plants used in French folk medicine included lavender, chamomile, rosemary, thyme, vervain, and many others.

Traditional Recipes: French folk healing relied on traditional recipes and formulations passed down through generations. These recipes involved specific combinations of herbs, roots, and other ingredients. Each remedy was believed to address specific ailments or promote overall well-being. The precise recipes varied depending on the region and the knowledge of individual healers.

Infusions and Decoctions: Healing brews in France were often prepared as infusions or decoctions. Infusions involved steeping herbs in hot water for a period of time, while decoctions involved boiling the herbs in water to extract their medicinal properties. Both methods were used to create potent liquids that could be consumed as teas or tonics.

Local and Seasonal Ingredients: Witches and folk healers in France would utilize ingredients available in their local environment, taking advantage of the specific plants found in the region. They would gather herbs and flowers according to seasonal availability and their medicinal properties. Certain plants might be associated with specific seasons or festivals, and their use in healing brews would be aligned with those traditions.

Ritual and Intention: The preparation of healing brews often involved ritualistic practices and a focus on intention. Witches and folk healers believed that their intentions and energy infused into the brews would enhance their healing properties. Rituals might include incantations, invocations, or other symbolic actions to empower the healing brews with their intended effects.

Scottish Specifics

Herbal Knowledge: Witches and folk healers in Scotland possessed extensive knowledge of local plants and their medicinal properties. They would gather a variety of herbs, flowers, and other botanical ingredients for use in their healing brews. Common medicinal plants used in Scottish folk medicine included nettle, elderflower, bog myrtle, heather, yarrow, and many others.

Traditional Formulations: Scottish folk healing relied on traditional formulations and recipes passed down through generations. These formulations involved specific combinations of herbs, roots, and other ingredients, with each remedy believed to address specific ailments or promote general well-being. The exact recipes varied depending on the region and the knowledge of individual healers.

Infusions and Decoctions: Witches and folk healers in Scotland often prepared healing brews as infusions or decoctions. Infusions involved steeping herbs in hot water for a period of time, while decoctions involved boiling the herbs in water to extract their medicinal properties. Both methods were used to create potent liquids that could be consumed as teas or tonics.

Local and Wild Ingredients: Witches and folk healers in Scotland made use of ingredients available in their local environment, including those found in the Scottish countryside and Highlands. They gathered herbs and plants from their surroundings, taking advantage of their specific healing properties. This often included wild-growing plants, such as heather and bog myrtle.

Ritual and Folklore: The preparation of healing brews in Scotland often involved rituals and was intertwined with folklore and traditional practices. The use of chants, prayers, or other ritualistic elements was believed to enhance the healing properties of the brews. Folklore and cultural beliefs surrounding specific plants and rituals played a role in shaping the understanding of witches' healing abilities.

Cultural Differences between Witches in Germany, Switzerland, France and Scotland

There were cultural differences in the perception and practices associated with witches in Germany, Switzerland, France, and Scotland. These regional variations were influenced by factors such as historical events, religious beliefs, social norms, and local traditions.

Germany
In Germany, the perception of witches was often characterized by a blend of Christian beliefs, folklore, and traditional practices. Witches were commonly associated with harmful magic, malevolent activities, and causing misfortune. Accused witches were often feared and seen as threats to the community, resulting in witch trials and persecutions. However, Germany also had a strong tradition of wise women or folk healers who were respected for their knowledge of herbal remedies and practical healing techniques.

Switzerland
In Switzerland, the perception of witches varied depending on the region. Witches were believed to

possess both harmful and healing powers. Some witches were feared for their ability to inflict harm, while others were sought after for their knowledge of herbal remedies and practical healing techniques. Switzerland also had a tradition of wise women or folk healers who were respected for their healing skills. However, accusations of witchcraft often resulted in persecution due to the association of their practices with malevolent magic.

France
In France, the perception of witches evolved over time. Witches were increasingly associated with harmful practices, malevolent activities, and pacts with supernatural entities. The perception of witches as healers diminished, and their alleged healing powers were often disregarded or interpreted as part of their malevolent activities. The influence of the Catholic Church played a significant role in shaping the perception of witches and their association with witchcraft trials.

Scotland
In Scotland, the perception of witches had a distinctive cultural context. Scotland had a tradition of cunning folk or wise women who were respected for their healing abilities. These women played a crucial role in providing remedies, midwifery services, and practical healing techniques to their communities. While

accusations of witchcraft and witch trials also occurred in Scotland, there was a greater recognition and acceptance of certain healing practices associated with witches.

These cultural differences highlight the diverse ways in which witchcraft was perceived and understood within different regions. The beliefs, practices, and societal attitudes towards witches and their healing abilities varied, influenced by factors such as religious traditions, social structures, and historical events.

Witches Brews and Modern Day Medicine

The concept of witches' brews from historical times and modern-day medicine are not directly related. However, it's important to note that traditional folk healing practices, including the use of herbs and natural remedies, have influenced certain aspects of modern herbal medicine and complementary and alternative medicine (CAM).

In the past, witches' brews were often associated with folk remedies, herbal concoctions, and traditional healing practices. These brews were made from various plants, herbs, and other ingredients believed to possess medicinal properties. While some of these historical practices were based on traditional knowledge and folklore, others may have had limited effectiveness or relied on superstition.

In modern times, evidence-based medicine and scientific research play a central role in determining the safety and efficacy of medical treatments. Modern medicine focuses on rigorous scientific methods, clinical trials, and regulatory standards to evaluate the benefits and potential risks of pharmaceuticals and medical interventions.

However, it is worth noting that there is a resurgence of interest in herbal medicine and complementary approaches to health and wellness. Some traditional remedies and herbal preparations have found their place within modern herbal medicine and CAM practices. The use of herbal infusions, tinctures, and extracts made from specific plants and herbs is still prevalent in certain contexts.

Modern herbal medicine incorporates scientific research and evidence-based approaches to understand the chemical components and potential therapeutic effects of plants and herbs. Some traditional remedies have been studied and validated for their medicinal properties, leading to the development of standardized herbal preparations and supplements.

Witchcraft vs. today's Pharmaceutical Industry

The approaches to healing associated with witches in historical times were significantly different from the practices and principles of today's pharmaceutical industry.

Beliefs and Worldview: Witches' approach to healing was often intertwined with supernatural or magical beliefs. They believed in the power of spells, charms, and rituals to influence health and well-being. Their practices were rooted in folk traditions, ancient beliefs, and spiritual or metaphysical concepts.

Methods and Ingredients: Witches' healing practices involved the use of natural remedies, such as herbal infusions, poultices, and salves, often prepared from plants and other ingredients available in their local environments. These remedies were based on traditional knowledge and sometimes included elements of folk wisdom, superstitions, and cultural beliefs. In contrast, the pharmaceutical industry claims to utilize sophisticated laboratory research and technology to identify, isolate, and synthesize specific chemical compounds that have demonstrated therapeutic effects. These compounds are then formulated into pharmaceutical drugs that undergo rigorous testing, regulation, and quality control.

Efficacy and Safety: The efficacy and safety of witches' healing practices varied and were often based on cultural beliefs, traditions, and personal experiences. While some natural remedies used by witches may have had beneficial effects, others could be ineffective or even harmful.

Professionalism and Standards: Witches' healing practices were often carried out by individuals within local communities who possessed knowledge and skills passed down through generations. Their practices lacked the formal training, scientific understanding, and standardized protocols found in modern healthcare systems. In contrast, the pharmaceutical industry operates within a professional framework with stringent regulations, quality control measures, and ethical guidelines. Thousands of drugs have been recalled though.

While there are clear differences between witches' approaches to healing and the pharmaceutical industry, it's important to note that the historical practices of witches were rooted in their cultural and historical contexts.

Skin in the Game

Witches faced severe consequences, including persecution, if their healing practices were perceived as going wrong or if they were accused of wrongdoing. The social, cultural, and political contexts of the time often contributed to the persecution and marginalization of individuals associated with witchcraft.

In contrast, the modern pharmaceutical industry operates within a complex framework of regulations, quality control measures, and oversight. The development, testing, and approval of drugs involve extensive clinical trials, scientific research, and regulatory processes to assess their benefits and risks. Government agencies, such as the Food and Drug Administration (FDA) in the United States or the European Medicines Agency (EMA) in the European Union, play a vital role in the regulation and approval of pharmaceutical products.

While modern pharmaceutical companies may face legal and regulatory consequences if their products are found to be unsafe or ineffective, the responsible people usually got no skin in the game and suffer no personal consequences.

The consequences faced by individuals associated with the historical practice of witchcraft, including healing, were severe and often life-threatening. Accusations of witchcraft could lead to persecution, torture, and execution, with individuals facing personal consequences for their alleged actions.

It's important to recognize that historical witchcraft accusations and the consequences associated with them were often based on superstition, fear, and societal beliefs, rather than objective evidence or a fair legal system. The severity and personal nature of the consequences faced by accused witches were a product of the social and cultural context of the time.

Modern day pharmaceutical industry works like this: According to the FDA there are 955 drugs listed as "Recalls, Market Withdrawals, & Safety Alerts" 02/08/2018 - 07/12/2023.

www.ingramcontent.com/pod-product-compliance
Lightning Source LLC
Chambersburg PA
CBHW061404160726
47995CB00001B/450